TETANUS

PREVENTIVE PROCESSES OF TETANUS

DR. AHMED .R.

Contents

CHAPTER ONE

Definition

An extremely painful bacterial disease called tetanus affects your nervous system and causes painful muscle contractions, especially in the muscles of your neck and jaw. Tetanus can make it difficult for you to breathe, which could ultimately be fatal. One common name for tetanus is "lockjaw."

Tetanus cases are uncommon in the developed world, including the United States, because of the tetanus vaccine. Less developed nations have far higher tetanus incidence rates. Globally, there are about a million cases reported annually.

Tetanus cannot be cured. The goal of treatment is to manage complications while the tetanus toxin's effects subside. The highest rates of death are seen in those who are not immunized and in older adults who have received insufficient vaccinations.

After tetanus bacteria enter your body through a wound, signs and symptoms of the disease can manifest anywhere from a few days to several weeks later. Seven to eight days are the typical incubation period.

In the following order of appearance, common tetanus signs and symptoms are:

Your jaw muscles are tense and in spasms.

Your neck muscles are stiff.

Swallowing difficulties

Tenseness in your lower abdomen

Excruciating body spasms that last for several minutes and are usually brought on by insignificant events like a draft, a loud noise, a physical touch, or light

Additional indications and symptoms could be:

Temperature spike

Perspiring

Increased blood pressure

Elevated heart rate

When to consult a physician

If you have a deep or dirty wound, have not received a tetanus booster shot in the last five years, or are unsure when you last received one, see your doctor to get a booster shot. If you haven't received a tetanus booster in the last ten years or are unsure of when you received your last vaccination, you should speak with your doctor about getting one for any wound, particularly if it has been exposed to manure, animal feces, or dirt.

The reasons

Dust, soil, and animal excrement all contain Clostridium tetani, the bacteria that causes tetanus. The bacteria can release a potent toxin called tetanospasmin when they penetrate a deep flesh wound. This toxin actively damages the motor neurons in your body, which are the nerves that regulate your muscles. Tetanus symptoms such as muscle stiffness and spasms are primarily caused by the toxin's effect on your motor neurons.

Hazard elements

Furthermore, for the tetanus bacteria to multiply in your body, a few conditions must be met. Among these are:

Inadequate or nonexistent tetanus vaccination, which includes missing booster shots on time

A penetration-related wound that allows tetanus spores to enter the wound

Additional pathogenic bacteria present

Damaged tissue

Something foreign, like a splinter or nail

Swelling in the vicinity of the wound

The following injury types have resulted in tetanus cases:

injuries from punctures, such as those caused by splinters, body piercings, tattoos, and injection drugs

Gunshot injuries

Fractures of compound nature

Crush wounds

Burns

Incisions from surgery

Injection drug usage

Infections in the ears

Bites from animals

Foot ulcers that are infected

Newborns with insufficient immunizations exhibiting infected umbilical stumps

CHAPTER TWO

Complications

It is impossible to get rid of tetanus toxin once it has attached itself to your nerve endings. The development of new nerve endings is necessary for full recovery from a tetanus infection, and this process may take several months.

Among the potential tetanus infection complications are:

Bones broken. The vertebrae and other bones may fracture due to the intensity of spasms.

incapacity. Strong sedatives are usually used to manage muscle spasms during tetanus treatment.

The use of these medications can cause prolonged immobility, which can result in permanent disability. Tetanus infections in infants have the potential to cause permanent brain damage, varying from mild mental impairments to cerebral palsy.

Demise. You may experience periods of complete dyspnea if you suffer from severe tetanus-induced (tetanic) muscle spasms. The most frequent reason for death is respiratory failure. A deficiency of oxygen can also result in cardiac arrest and death. Another reason for demise is pneumonia.

Start by visiting your family doctor if your wound is clean and small but you're worried about infection or whether you're immune to tetanus. Seek emergency medical attention if the wound is severe or if you or your child is exhibiting signs of a tetanus infection.

What's at your disposal?

If at all feasible, kindly give your doctor the information below:

When, where, and how you were hurt (or, if a wound isn't visible, any recent injury)

A documentation of the vaccinations you have got and when they were administered would be beneficial. Your immunization status, including the date of your most recent tetanus booster shot

How have you been tending to the wound?

Any long-term medical conditions you may already have, such as diabetes, heart disease, or pregnancy

Inform the physician about the mother's immigration history, her immune system, and the length of time she has lived in the United States if you are seeking care for a baby who is not your own.

What's the greatest thing to do?

What are the alternatives that you provide to the main strategy?

These are the additional medical ailments I have. How can I co-manage them?

Should I consult an expert?

Do I have to abide by any restrictions?

Does the medication you're recommending have a generic counterpart?

Are there any printed materials available for me to carry with me, such as brochures? Which websites are you recommending?

Your doctor will examine any visible wounds. It is probable that they will pose several inquiries to you, such as:

When did the symptoms of tentanus begin to appear if you have had any?

Have your symptoms been constant or sporadic?

What degree of severity do you have symptoms of?

What seems to help or aggravate your issues, if anything?

What kind of vaccine and when was your most recent tetanus vaccination?

If it's not evident, have you suffered any wounds recently?

Exams as well as diagnosis

In addition to a physical examination, a patient's medical and immunization history, and the signs and symptoms of pain, stiffness, and spasming muscles, doctors diagnose tetanus. For the most part, laboratory testing is not useful in diagnosing tetanus.

MEDICATION AND DRUG USE

Tetanus has no known cure; therefore, supportive care, painkillers, and wound care are the mainstays of treatment.

Wound healing

To stop tetanus spores from growing, the wound must be cleaned. This is cleaning the wound of debris, dead tissue, and foreign things.

Drugs

Antitoxin. A tetanus antitoxin, such as tetanus immune globulin, may be prescribed by your physician. But the antitoxin can only counteract toxins that haven't yet attached themselves to nerve tissue.

drugs known as antibiotics. Antibiotics, administered orally or via injection, may also be prescribed by your physician to combat tetanus bacteria.

vaccine. You remain susceptible to the bacterium even after being tetanus-positive once. To avoid contracting tetanus in the future, you must therefore get vaccinated against the disease.

Adrenaline. To manage muscle spasms, doctors typically employ strong sedatives.

other medications. To help control involuntary muscle activity, such your heartbeat and respiration, additional drugs like magnesium sulfate and certain beta blockers may be prescribed. In addition to sedation, morphine can be utilized for this.

Supportive treatment

Treatment for tetanus infection in a critical care unit typically takes a long time. You might require temporary ventilator support since sedatives might cause shallow breathing.

HOME RECOGNITION AND LIFESTYLE

Being inoculated against the toxin makes tetanus easily preventable. Most tetanus cases happen to persons who have never received an immunization or who have not received a booster dose in the ten years prior.

The first vaccination series

The diphtheria and tetanus toxoids and acellular pertussis (DTaP) vaccine often includes the tetanus shot. This immunization offers defense against whooping cough (pertussis), tetanus, and a throat and respiratory infection (diphtheria).

The DTaP vaccine is administered to children in the arm or thigh, usually over the course of five injections, at the following ages:

Two months

Four months

half a year

15–18 months

4–6 years

The uplift

Tetanus booster shots are usually administered in conjunction with diphtheria booster shots (Td).

A tetanus, diphtheria, and pertussis (Tdap) vaccination was authorized in 2005 for use in adults and teenagers under the age of 65 in order to guarantee ongoing protection against pertussis.

Teenagers should have a Tdap dose, ideally between the ages of 11 and 12, and after that, they should receive a Td booster every ten years. Replace the Tdap dose with your subsequent Td booster dose if you have never gotten one, and then keep receiving Td boosters.

If you are going abroad, it is advisable to have a current vaccination record because tetanus cases could be higher there, particularly in underdeveloped nations. Get another booster shot if it has been more than five years since your last one and you sustain a serious or dirty wound.

See your doctor frequently to have your immunization status reviewed in order to ensure that you are up to date on all of your shots.

Discuss receiving the Tdap vaccination with your doctor if you were not given a tetanus vaccination as a youngster.

THE END